W9-DHT-961

WE CAN SAVE THE EARTH

HEALTHY EARTH,
HEALTHY BODIES

Written by:
Jill C. Wheeler

Published by Abdo & Daughters, 6535 Cecilia Circle, Edina, Minnesota 55439.

Library bound edition distributed by Rockbottom Books, Pentagon Tower, P.O. Box 36036, Minneapolis, Minnesota 55435.

Library of Congress Number: 91-073069   ISBN: 1-56239-032-5

Cover Illustrations by: C.A. Nobens
Interiors by: Kristi Schaeppi

Edited by: Stuart Kallen

TABLE OF CONTENTS

Introduction..4

Chapter 1..**8**
Dangerous Metals

Chapter 2...**12**
Chemical Contaminants

Chapter 3...**17**
When Energy Kills

Chapter 4...**24**
What You Can Do

A Final Note...**30**

Glossary..**32**

INTRODUCTION

In 1974, the Three Mile Island Nuclear Power Plant in Harrisburg, Pennsylvania, began generating electricity. The company that built the plant said it was a breakthrough in energy production. They said that the nuclear power plant would not create pollution like power plants that burned fossil fuels.

Yet strange things began to happen near the new plant. Within two years of its opening, local farmers noticed their animals were behaving strangely. Many of the animals would fall down for no reason. Many baby animals, including calves, kittens and ducklings, were born deformed or dead. The farmers said that they had never had so many sick animals before.

People noticed other strange things as well. There were not as many wild birds, squirrels and rabbits as there used to be. Many trees died and others were losing their bark. Something was wrong.

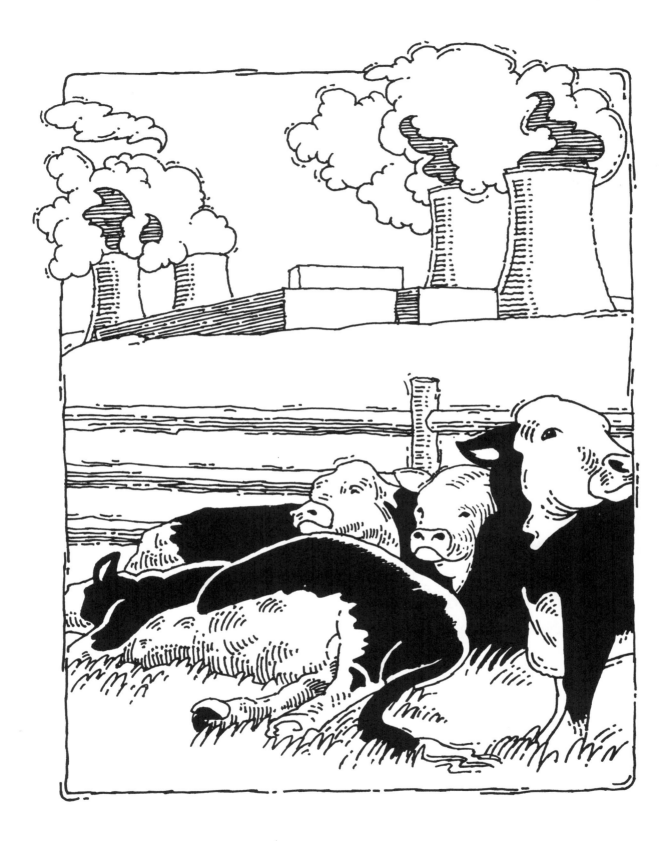

That something turned out to be the power plant. And when the plant malfunctioned in March 1979, the problems increased. Even more animals got sick and died.

Scientists often look at animals to see how a substance will affect people. Because animals are smaller and have shorter life spans, things that can harm people will first show up in animals. In that way, people learned that the radiation from the Three Mile Island plant that had made the animals sick would make them sick too. They were able to prevent the plant from reopening after the accident.

As you can see, we have many things in common with the plants and animals who share the Earth with us. We all are living organisms. We all need the air, the water and the land to survive. When anything happens to the Earth, it affects all of us.

The Earth today is much different than it was just 100 years ago. In many ways the Earth is sicker because people have polluted it. Just as the pollution has made the Earth sick, it is also making more and more people sick. Things that make people sick are called toxins.

In this book, we will look at how a sick Earth can create sick people. We'll see how the things we've done to the air, the water and the land have come back to haunt us. We will also find out what things we can do to protect ourselves while we nurse the Earth – and ourselves – back to health.

Did You Know...

- According to the International Atomic Energy Agency, a major nuclear accident is likely to occur every 10 years.

- In 1971, cancer killed 337,000 people a year. In 1986, it killed 472,000.

- Between 1970 and 1985, 18 of the 27 most common birth defects increased in incidence, some as much as 1,700%.

CHAPTER 1

Dangerous Metals

When you think of metal, you probably think of cars, cans and other things that are made from metal. But people also have some metals inside their bodies.

The healthy human body needs metals such as copper and iron to function properly. But like any substance, too much copper or iron can make a person sick. Pollution causes many types of poisonous metals to enter the human body. These poisonous metals include lead, aluminum, cadmium, and mercury.

Lead is among the worst of unhealthy metals. Lead is found in many things including paints, water pipes and auto exhaust. People who are around lead pollution for long periods of time can get too much lead in their bodies. The lead gets into their blood through food and water, as well as the air they breathe. This is called lead poisoning.

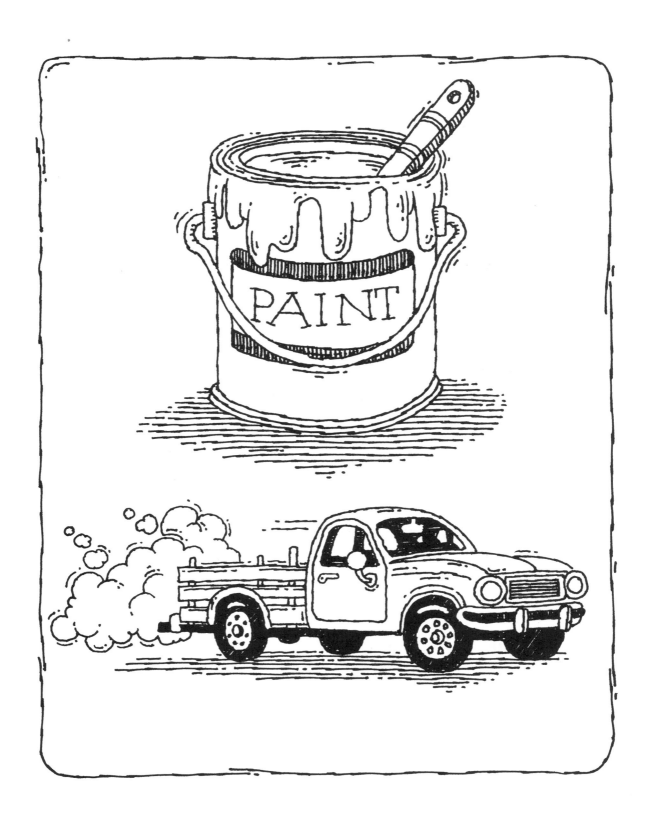

As the lead builds up in the human body, people experience many different problems. Common effects of lead poisoning include learning disabilities, especially in children, high blood pressure, hearing loss, and brain damage.

Aluminum can also make people sick. Scientists have discovered that aluminum cookware and aluminum foil can transfer aluminum into food, which is then ingested into the body. Too much aluminum can lead to intestinal problems, hardening of the arteries, and Alzheimer's disease. People with Alzheimer's disease lose their memory and often do not know where they are.

Cadmium is produced during the burning of fossil fuels such as oil and coal. Cadmium compounds also are used to make plastics and batteries. Too much cadmium in a person's body often leads to kidney disease and lung damage. It also can hurt unborn babies.

Mercury is another metal that can be poisonous to humans. In the late 1950s, people living near Minamata Bay in Japan began to suffer from a strange disease. Many of the children born to people in the area had birth defects, others had mental disabilities. It was discovered the people were sick because a local factory had been dumping wastes into the bay. The wastes contained mercury. The people got sick when they ate fish that had swallowed the waste.

Metals are just some of the many pollutants that harm people and the Earth. Perhaps even more harmful are some of the chemicals being used in the 1990s. The next chapter looks at some of those chemicals and their effects on our health.

Did You Know...
- More than 2,100 chemical contaminants were found in U.S. public water systems between 1971 and 1985.

- Pesticide contamination of the food supply may be responsible for up to 20,000 cancer cases each year.

- Americans suffer 20 to 90 million cases of illness due to food contamination each year.

CHAPTER 2

Chemical Contaminants

There are more than seven million known chemicals, and thousands more are being developed every year. These chemicals are used for everything from cleaning to killing insects on crops to manufacturing plastics.

Chemicals have made our lives easier in many ways. They have also made our environment more deadly by contaminating our air and water. In the 1970s for example, scientists found more than 700 chemical compounds in the drinking water in Cincinnati, Ohio.

Not all chemicals cause sickness, but some have been identified as being extremely hazardous to human health. Among these are polychlorinated biphenyls (pol-ee-klor-ah-nat-ed bi-fen-els), or PCBs; a group of substances called Volatile Organic Chemicals, or VOCs; nitrates and sulfates.

PCBs are oily, synthetic chemicals that have been widely used since the 1930s. Because PCBs do not easily burn or corrode, they are useful in the production of electrical products. They also are used in the manufacture of air conditioners, refrigerators, television sets and paints. PCBs have a very stable chemical makeup, so they are difficult to destroy. As a result, once they are burned or buried in landfills, PCBs do not disappear. They escape to the air, water or soil.

Once in the environment, PCBs contaminate plants, which are ingested by animals. Humans are contaminated with PCBs when they eat contaminated fish, animals, or animal products. In Montana the PCBs that leaked out of one electrical transformer contaminated livestock and human food in 17 states.

For many years, PCBs have been known to make people sick. But the real hazards of PCBs did not come to light until more than one thousand people were poisoned by them in Japan in 1968. It was then that people realized that PCBs could cause humans to become tired and sick to their stomachs, or cause their livers to be damaged.

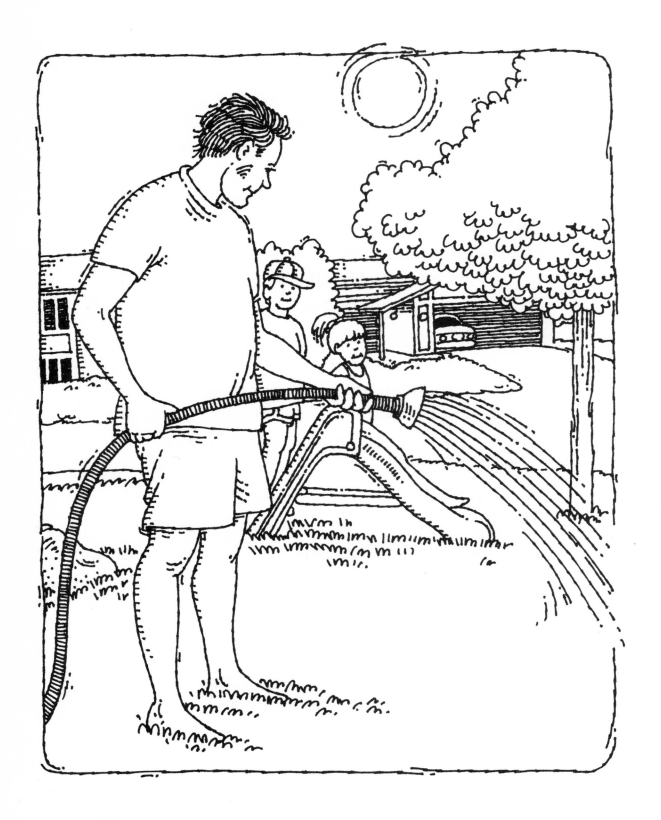

VOCs are a family of chemical solvents. A solvent is a substance that can dissolve or disperse another chemical. VOCs are widely used in cleaning and removing grease from metals, as well as for dry-cleaning. These chemicals often are found in the water, but they easily enter the air. People can inhale or absorb VOCs into their skin by showering with, boiling, or just using VOC-contaminated water.

Once in the body, VOCs may lead to memory loss, damage to the immune system (which protects us from disease), kidney damage, and cancer. Cancer occurs when damaged cells multiply more rapidly than good cells.

Nitrates are chemicals that primarily come from synthetic fertilizers spread on farm fields and lawns. Most nitrate pollution is in the water, although nitrates are also found in the air. In humans, nitrates reduce the amount of oxygen in the blood. This can be deadly, especially for babies. Nitrates also can cause birth defects involving the spinal cord.

Sulfates are found in the air. When fossil fuels such as coal and oil are burned, sulfur dioxide is created. Sulfur dioxide then changes into sulfates.

15

Particles of sulfates carry sulfuric acid and other toxic chemicals into the lungs. There, they irritate the respiratory system, causing illnesses such as asthma, bronchitis and emphysema. Researchers estimate that sulfates are responsible for the deaths of 100,000 people each year. Sulfates also have been linked to cancer.

PCBs, VOCs, nitrates and sulfates are just a few of the many chemicals which are hurting both the Earth and the people who live on it. Another invisible, yet deadly pollutant is also stalking people around the world. In the next chapter, we'll see how people are dying from something they can't see, touch, taste or even smell.

Did You Know...
- The explosion at the Chernobyl reactor released 90 times the radiation of the nuclear bomb dropped on Hiroshima, Japan in 1945.

CHAPTER 3

When Energy Kills

On April 26, 1986, the nuclear reactor at Chernobyl in the Soviet Union blew up, releasing one-tenth of the reactor's radioactivity. It was the worst industrial accident in the history of the world.

The accident scattered radiation for hundreds of miles around the reactor. Radiation is the name for a family of energy forms that includes light, heat rays, ultraviolet rays, x-rays, gamma rays and radio waves. Some of those rays, such as ultraviolet rays, x-rays, and gamma rays can make people sick.

More than 135,000 people who lived near the Chernobyl reactor were forced to leave their homes. Others stayed, unaware that their bodies had been contaminated by radiation.

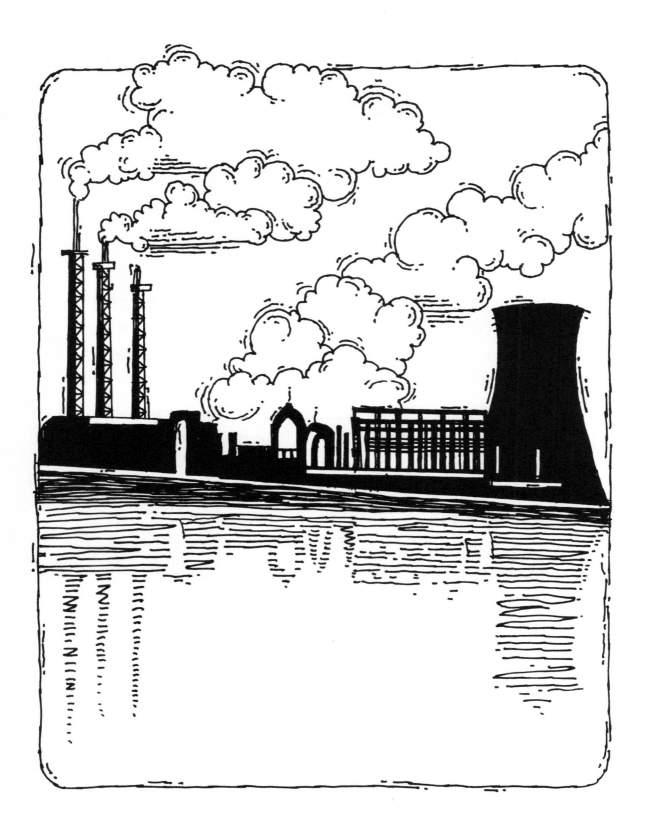

The accident affected other parts of the world, too. Radioactive fallout was carried by the winds to Great Britain, France, and even the United States. Humans, animals and food sources all were contaminated.

The Chernobyl reactor is just one of hundreds of nuclear power plants that have been built around the world. Nuclear power was first developed in the United States in the early 1940s to provide a new source of energy.

Nuclear power involves splitting a uranium atom into two almost equal parts. This process, called fission, happens inside the nuclear reactor. When the atom is split, it generates huge amounts of heat and creates a chain reaction to split other atoms. Temperatures in nuclear reactors can reach more than 500 degrees Fahrenheit.

The heat from the chain reaction is used to boil water, and the steam from the boiling water is run through turbines, creating electricity. The electricity is used by people to light their homes and offices, cook their food and run their appliances.

When it first was developed, nuclear power was hailed as a way to produce the electricity people needed without having to burn fossil fuels. It was said that with nuclear power, the air would not be polluted as it is by burning fossil fuels. In addition, people would never run out of the materials needed to produce nuclear power, while fossil fuels cannot be replaced once they are gone.

But nuclear reactors also produce radiation. The radiation leaks out into the environment when the water used to cool the reactor is dumped outside as waste water. Radiation also can escape through reactor plant smokestacks. Even if no accidents occur, some radiation always escapes.

The spent fuel rods from nuclear power plants remain highly toxic for tens of thousands of years. No safe way has been found to store these poisons forever.

Radiation makes people sick by attacking the cells of their bodies. The cell is the most basic element of all living organisms. Cells take in food, get rid of wastes, produce protein necessary for life, and reproduce. There are more than 10 trillion cells in the human body.

Radioactive particles can penetrate cells and either kill or damage them. If a damaged cell cannot repair itself before it reproduces, the damage is repeated in another cell, and another, and so on.

One of the worst ways radiation hurts people is when the radioactive particle damages the DNA in a cell. DNA, or deoxyribonucleic acid, is a "blueprint" that tells the cell what to do. Radiation can change the DNA so it tells the cell to become something different than it should be. That cell then divides to form other damaged cells.

When there are thousands of damaged cells, people get tumors. As these bad cells multiply, they take over body parts which used to be made up of normal cells. This is called cancer.

Cancer can occur in many human organs. Some organs which tend to develop cancer because of exposure to radiation are the pancreas, the lungs, the large intestine, the thyroid, and the liver.

Radiation also leads to many other illnesses, including pneumonia, tuberculosis, vision problems such as cataracts and anemia, other blood disorders, headaches, sleeplessness, nosebleeds, and hair loss. Not all symptoms occur immediately. Some, like tumors and leukemia, show up after three or four years. Genetic disorders appear in the next generation.

The use of fossil fuels has also increased the amount of radiation on Earth. Carbon dioxide and nitrogen dioxide produced by burning fossil fuels has been eating away at the Earth's protective ozone layer. The ozone is an invisible layer of gas which shields the Earth from many of the sun's ultraviolet rays. Ultraviolet rays are a form of radiation. Too much ultraviolet radiation can cause people to develop cancer.

Even though we cannot see radiation, there are things we can do to protect ourselves from its effects. In the next chapter, we'll look at what we can do to stay healthy while living on a poisoned planet.

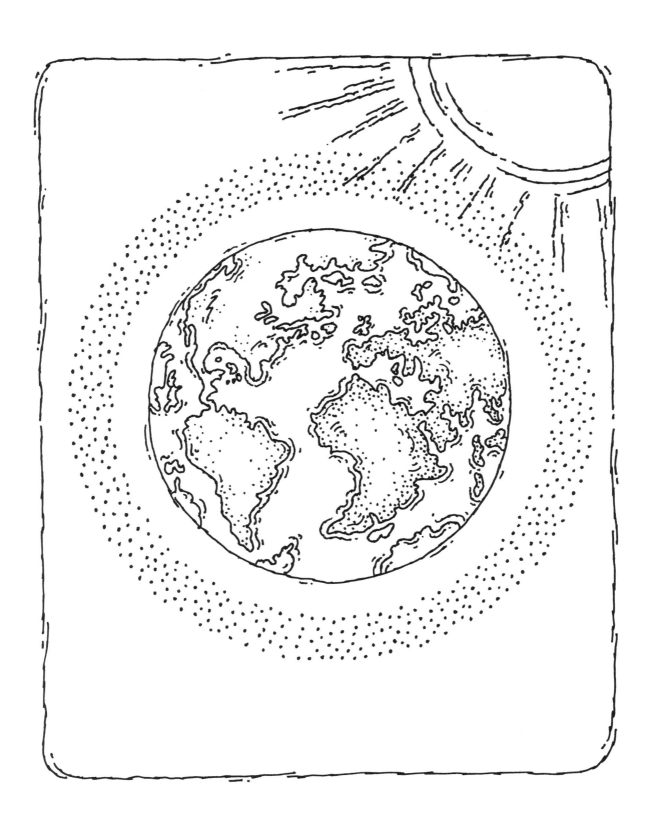

CHAPTER 4

What You Can Do

If we want healthy bodies, we must first create a healthy earth. Many people are working to do that right now through recycling, energy conservation, wildlife preservation, waste reduction and the elimination of harmful chemicals.

It has taken many years for the Earth to become as polluted as it is now. And it will take many years to nurse it back to health.

In the meantime, there are steps you and your family can take to stay healthy. Here are some ideas:

De-Toxify Yourself!

• Avoid aluminum! Ask your parents to stop using aluminum cookware. Have them use waxed paper to cover foods instead of aluminum foil. Look on the labels of antacids, buffered pain killers, table salt and convenience foods. If the products contain aluminum, don't use them.

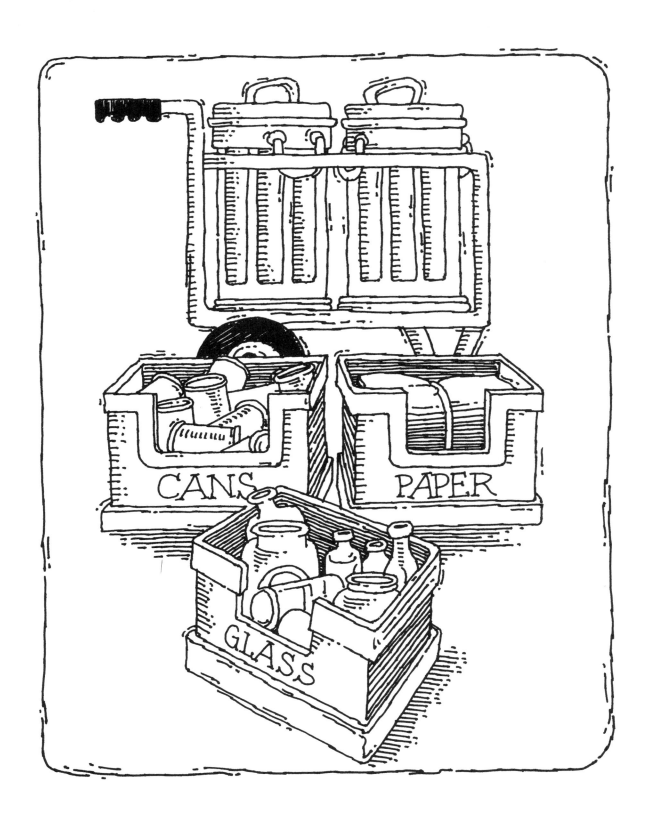

- Eat plenty of grains, beans, and vegetables. These plants are low on the food chain so they contain fewer toxins. Food from animals contains a much higher percentage of toxins. These toxins build up in the animals' bodies from the pesticides and growth hormones in the food they eat. Farm animals also absorb toxins from fertilizer run-off in the water they drink and pollution in the air they breathe.

- Drink lots of clean water. Water helps get toxins out of the body. So does sweating.

- If you live in an older home with lead-soldered pipes, draw your drinking water at the end of the day when the lead levels are lower. Use water drawn first thing in the morning for cleaning, doing dishes or watering plants.

- Beware of eating food or water from glazed ceramic pottery. Many pieces of pottery contain toxic cadmium or lead in their glaze. The toxins can be transferred to any food that is stored in them or eaten from them. Pottery made in Mexico, Spain, Italy, Portugal, China and Korea should be avoided. Use it for plants or for decoration, instead.

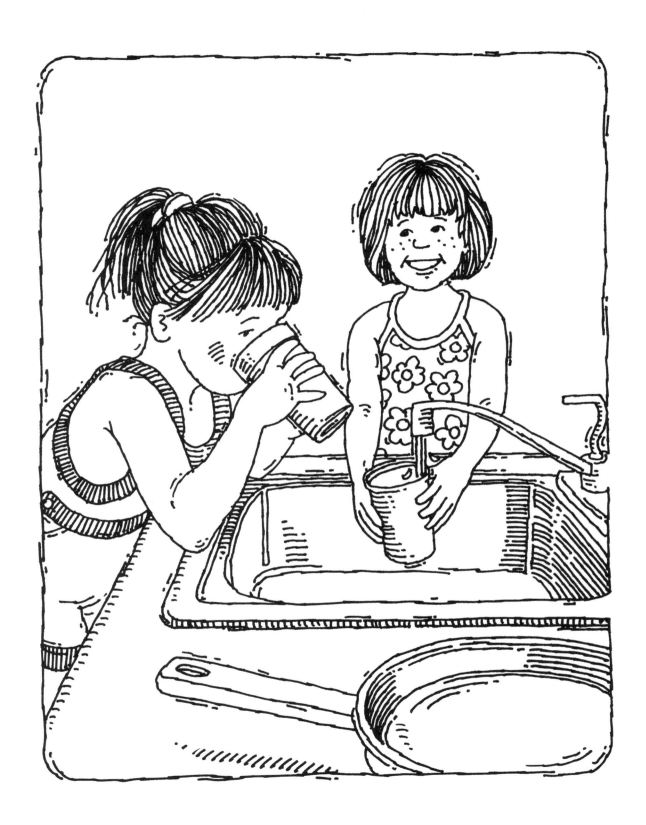

- Choose organically grown produce whenever possible. Organic means no chemicals were used to grow it.

- Remove your shoes before going into your house. The dust on your shoes may contain lead from automobile exhaust.

- Always wash your hands before eating. Your hands can pick up contaminants from the air and the things you touch.

- Urge your parents to use nontoxic substitutes for household cleaners. Vinegar, baking soda and borax are good substitutes.

- Write to your elected officials and urge them to invest in energy sources other than fossil fuels and nuclear energy. These include solar, wind and thermal energy. Encourage them to step up energy conservation measures too.

- Ask your parents to have your drinking water analyzed. If it is unsafe, buy bottled drinking water or install a good water purification system.

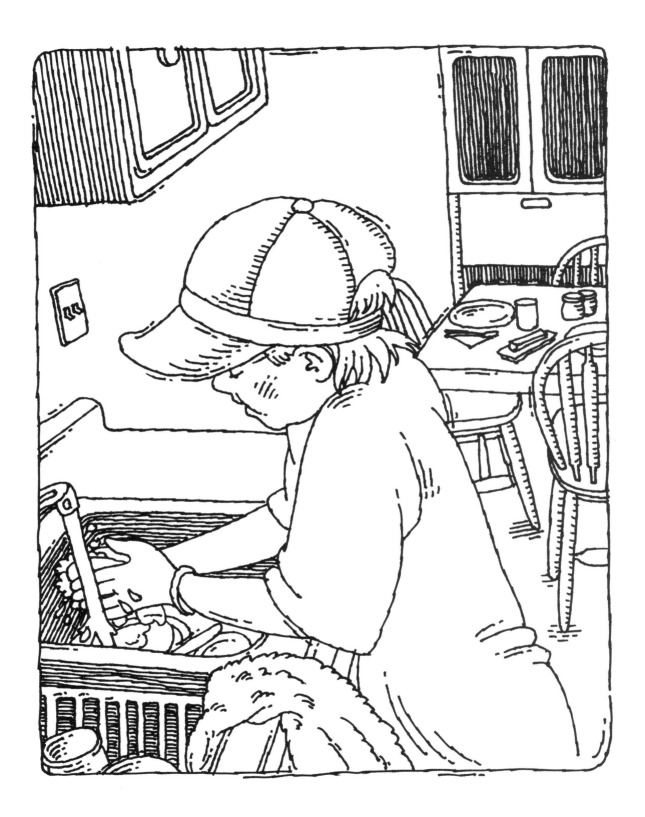

A FINAL NOTE

In the United States, there are several governmental agencies whose job it is to make sure people are not exposed to toxic substances. These agencies work with researchers to determine how much of these substances are too much. They determine how much of a substance a person can tolerate without getting sick. This amount, called an acceptable level, is used to regulate the use of the substance.

Unfortunately, there are problems with this system. For example, one government agency determining acceptable levels of pesticides assumes people only consume residue from that one pesticide. They do not consider that people eat foods containing residues from hundreds of different pesticides. While people may never eat enough of any one pesticide to get sick, they may get sick from eating tiny amounts of many different pesticides.

The same is true of other contaminants like metals, radiation and other chemicals. Alone, they are harmless. But when piled on each other in the body, they cause problems.

Some people are telling the government it must be more careful about determining acceptable levels of contaminants. You can do the same by writing to your elected officials and asking them to look at the effects of all contaminants, not just one.

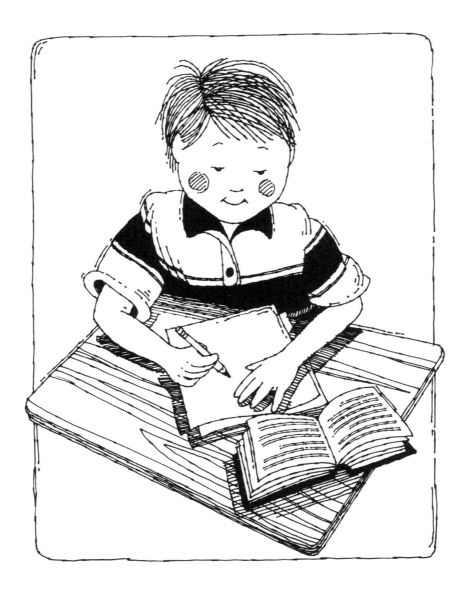

GLOSSARY

ATOM – The smallest particle of any substance.

CANCER – A disease in which body cells grow wildly.

GAMMA RAYS – A form of radiation. Gamma rays can penetrate living things and are used to make x-ray photographs.

LEUKEMIA – A disease that affects the parts of the body that make white blood cells.

RADIOACTIVITY – When a substance emits radiation in the form of alpha particles, beta particles or gamma rays.

SYNTHETIC – Something which does not occur in nature and is made only by people.

TUBERCULOSIS – A disease that usually affects the lungs.

URANIUM – A metallic chemical element used to fuel nuclear reactors.